RENAL DIET PLAN AND COOKBOOK

Renal Diet Cookbook for Newly Diagnosed Patients The Easy and Tasty Formula to Manage Early Stages of Kidney Disease and Avoid Dialysis

---

3

TABLE OF CONTENTS

—

BREAKFAST

Coconut Breakfast Smoothie

Preparation Time: 5 minutes

Cooking Time: 5 minutes

Servings: 1

Ingredients:

- 1/4 cup whey protein powder
- 1/2 cup coconut milk
- 5 drops liquid stevia
- 1 tbsp coconut oil
- 1 tsp vanilla
- 2 tbsp coconut butter
- 1/4 cup water
- 1/2 cup ice

Directions:

1. Add all ingredients into the blender and blend until smooth.
2. Serve and enjoy.

Nutrition: Calories 560 Fat 45 g Carbohydrates 12 g Sugar 4 g Protein 25 g Cholesterol 60 mg Phosphorus: 160mg Potassium: 127mg Sodium: 85mg

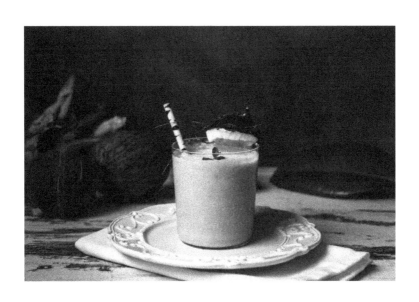

Turkey and Spinach Scramble on Melba Toast

Preparation Time: 5 minutes

Cooking Time: 15 minutes

Servings: 2

Ingredients:

- 1 tsp. Extra virgin olive oil
- 1 cup Raw spinach
- ½ clove, minced Garlic
- 1 tsp. grated Nutmeg
- 1 cup Cooked and diced turkey breast
- 4 slices Melba toast
- 1 tsp. Balsamic vinegar

Directions:

1. Heat a skillet over medium heat and add oil.
2. Add turkey and heat through for 6 to 8 minutes.
3. Add spinach, garlic, and nutmeg and stir-fry for 6 minutes more.
4. Plate up the Melba toast and top with spinach and turkey scramble.
5. Drizzle with balsamic vinegar and serve.

Nutrition: Calories: 301 Fat: 19g Carb: 12g Protein: 19g
Sodium: 360mg Potassium: 269mg Phosphorus: 215mg

Cheesy Scrambled Eggs with Fresh Herbs

Preparation Time: 15 minutes

Cooking Time: 10 minutes

Servings: 4

Ingredients:

- 3 Eggs
- 2 Egg whites
- ½ cup Cream cheese
- ¼ cup Unsweetened rice milk
- 1 tbsp. green part only Chopped scallion
- 1 tbsp. Chopped fresh tarragon
- 2 tbsps. Unsalted butter
- Ground black pepper to taste

Directions:

1. Whisk the eggs, egg whites, cream cheese, rice milk, scallions, and tarragon. Mix until smooth.
2. Melt the butter in a skillet.
3. Put egg mixture and cook for 5 minutes or until the eggs are thick and curds creamy.
4. Season with pepper and serve.

Nutrition: Calories: 221 Fat: 19g Carb: 3g Protein: 8g Sodium: 193mg Potassium: 140mg Phosphorus: 119mg

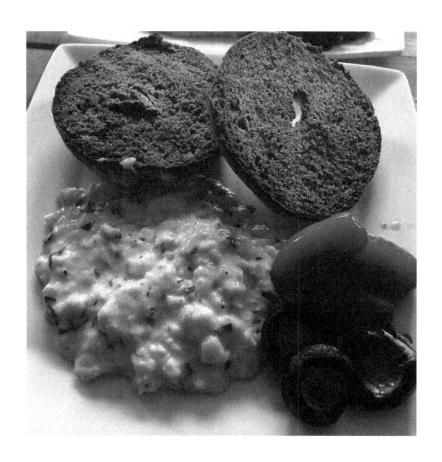

Mexican Style Burritos

Preparation Time: 5 minutes

Cooking Time: 15 minutes

Servings: 2

Ingredients:

- 1 tbsp. Olive oil
- 2 Corn tortillas
- ¼ cup chopped Red onion
- ¼ cup chopped Red bell peppers
- ½, deseeded and chopped red chili
- 2 Eggs
- 1 lime juice
- 1 tbsp. chopped Cilantro

Directions:

1. Place the tortillas in medium heat for 1 to 2 minutes on each side or until lightly toasted.

2. Remove and keep the broiler on.

3. Heat the oil in a skillet and sauté onion, chili, and bell peppers for 5 to 6 minutes or until soft.

4. Crack the eggs over the top of the onions and peppers.

5. Place skillet under the broiler for 5 to 6 minutes or until the eggs are cooked.

6. Serve half the eggs and vegetables on top of each tortilla and sprinkle with cilantro and lime juice to serve.

Nutrition: Calories: 202 Fat: 13g Carb: 19g Protein: 9g Sodium: 77mg Potassium: 233mg Phosphorus: 184mg

Bulgur, Couscous, and Buckwheat Cereal

Preparation Time: 10 minutes

Cooking Time: 25 minutes

Servings: 4

Ingredients:

- 2 ¼ cups Water
- 1 ¼ cups Vanilla rice milk
- 6 Tbsps. Uncooked bulgur
- 2 Tbsps. Uncooked whole buckwheat
- 1 cup Sliced apple
- 6 Tbsps. Plain uncooked couscous
- ½ tsp. Ground cinnamon

Directions:

1. Heat the water and milk in the saucepan over medium heat. Let it boil.

2. Put the bulgur, buckwheat, and apple.

3. Reduce the heat to low and simmer, occasionally stirring until the bulgur is tender, about 20 to 25 minutes.

4. Remove the saucepan and stir in the couscous and cinnamon—cover for 10 minutes.

5. Put the cereal before serving.

Nutrition: Calories: 159 Fat: 1g Carb: 34g Protein: 4g Sodium: 33mg Potassium: 116m Phosphorus: 130mg

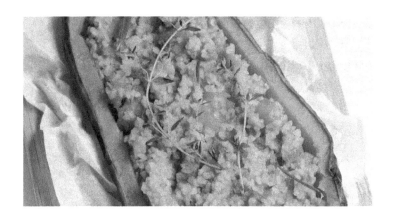

Blueberry Muffins

Preparation Time: 15 minutes

Cooking Time: 30 minutes

Servings: 12

Ingredients:

- 2 cups Unsweetened rice milk
- 1 Tbsp. Apple cider vinegar
- 3 ½ cups All-purpose flour
- 1 cup Granulated sugar
- 1 Tbsp. Baking soda substitute
- 1 tsp. Ground cinnamon
- ½ tsp. Ground nutmeg
- Pinch ground ginger
- ½ cup Canola oil
- 2 Tbsps. Pure vanilla extract
- 2 ½ cups Fresh blueberries

Directions:

1. Preheat the oven to 375F.
2. Prepare a muffin pan and set aside.
3. Stir together the rice milk and vinegar in a small bowl. Set aside for 10 minutes.

4. In a large bowl, stir together the sugar, flour, baking soda, cinnamon, nutmeg, and ginger until well mixed.

5. Add oil and vanilla to the milk and mix.

6. Put milk mixture to dry ingredients and stir well to combine.

7. Put the blueberries and spoon the muffin batter evenly into the cups.

8. Bake the muffins for 25 to 30 minutes or until golden and a toothpick inserted comes out clean.

9. Cool for 15 minutes and serve.

Nutrition: Calories: 331 Fat: 11g Carb: 52g Protein: 6g Sodium: 35mg Potassium: 89mg Phosphorus: 90mg

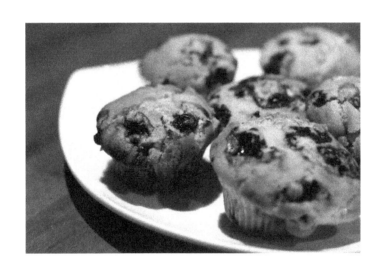

Buckwheat and Grapefruit Porridge

Preparation Time: 5 minutes

Cooking Time: 20 minutes

Servings: 2

Ingredients:

- ½ cup Buckwheat
- ¼ chopped Grapefruit
- 1 Tbsp. Honey
- 1 ½ cups Almond milk
- 2 cups Water

Directions:

1. Let the water boil on the stove. Add the buckwheat and place the lid on the pan.

2. Lower heat slightly and simmer for 7 to 10 minutes, checking to ensure water does not dry out.

3. When most of the water is absorbed, remove, and set aside for 5 minutes.

4. Drain any excess water from the pan and stir in almond milk, heating through for 5 minutes.

5. Add the honey and grapefruit.

6. Serve.

Nutrition: Calories: 231 Fat: 4g Carb: 43g Protein: 13g Sodium: 135mg Potassium: 370mg Phosphorus: 165mg

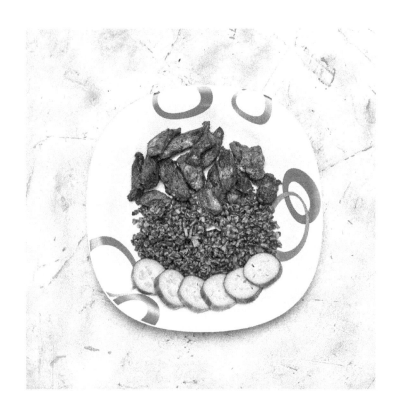

LUNCH

Arlecchino Rice Salad

Preparation Time: 10 minutes

Cooking Time: 15 minutes

Servings: 3

Ingredients:

- ½ cup white rice, dried
- 1 cup chicken stock
- 1 zucchini, shredded
- 2 tablespoons capers
- 1 carrot, shredded
- 1 tomato, chopped
- 1 tablespoon apple cider vinegar
- ½ teaspoon salt
- 2 tablespoons fresh parsley, chopped
- 1 tablespoon canola oil

Directions:

1. Put rice in the pan.
2. Add chicken stock and boil it with the closed lid for 15-20 minutes or until rice absorbs all water.
3. Meanwhile, in the mixing bowl combine together shredded zucchini, capers, carrot, and tomato.
4. Add fresh parsley.

5. Make the dressing: mix up together canola oil, salt, and apple cider vinegar.
6. Chill the cooked rice little and add it in the salad bowl to the vegetables.
7. Add dressing and mix up salad well.

Nutrition: calories 183, fat 5.3, fiber 2.1, carbs 30.4, protein 3.8
Phosphorus: 110mg Potassium: 117mg Sodium: 75mg

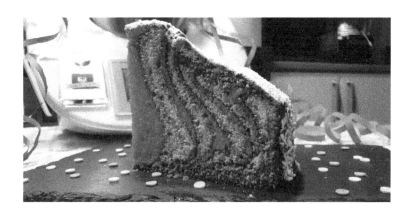

Sauteed Chickpea and Lentil Mix

Preparation Time: 10 minutes

Cooking Time: 50 minutes

Servings: 4

Ingredients:

- 1 cup chickpeas, half-cooked
- 1 cup lentils
- 5 cups chicken stock
- ½ cup fresh cilantro, chopped
- 1 teaspoon salt
- ½ teaspoon chili flakes
- ¼ cup onion, diced
- 1 tablespoon tomato paste

Directions:

1. Place chickpeas in the pan.
2. Add water, salt, and chili flakes.
3. Boil the chickpeas for 30 minutes over the medium heat.
4. Then add diced onion, lentils, and tomato paste. Stir well.
5. Close the lid and cook the mix for 15 minutes.
6. After this, add chopped cilantro, stir the meal well and cook it for 5 minutes more.
7. Let the cooked lunch chill little before serving.

Nutrition: calories 370, fat 4.3, fiber 23.7, carbs 61.6, protein 23.2 Phosphorus: 110mg Potassium: 117mg Sodium: 75mg

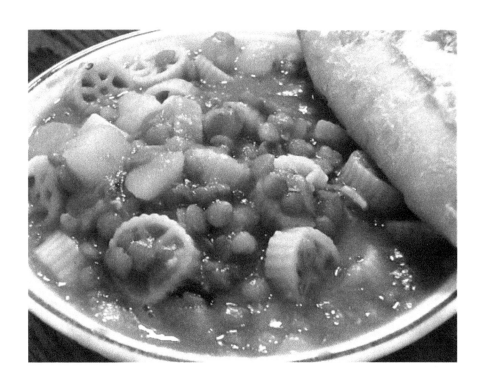

Crazy Japanese Potato and Beef Croquettes

Preparation Time: 10 minutes

Cooking Time: 20 minutes

Servings: 10

Ingredients:

- 3 medium russet carrots, peeled and chopped
- 1 tablespoon almond butter
- 1 tablespoon vegetable oil
- 3 onions, diced
- ¾ pound ground beef
- 4 teaspoons light coconut aminos
- All-purpose flour for coating
- 2 eggs, beaten
- Panko bread crumbs for coating
- ½ cup oil, frying

Directions:

1. Take a saucepan and place it over medium-high heat; add carrots and sunflower seeds water, boil for 16 minutes.
2. Remove water and put carrots in another bowl, add almond butter and mash the carrots.
3. Take a frying pan and place it over medium heat, add 1 tablespoon oil and let it heat up.
4. Add onions and stir fry until tender.
5. Add coconut aminos to beef to onions.
6. Keep frying until beef is browned.
7. Mix the beef with the carrots evenly.

8. Take another frying pan and place it over medium heat; add half a cup of oil.
9. Form croquettes using the mashed potato mixture and coat them with flour, then eggs and finally breadcrumbs.
10. Fry patties until golden on all sides.
11. Enjoy!

Nutrition: Calories: 239 Fat: 4g Carbohydrates: 20g Protein: 10g Phosphorus: 120mg Potassium: 107mg Sodium: 75mg

Traditional Black Bean Chili

Preparation Time: 10 minutes

Cooking Time: 4 hours

Servings: 4

Ingredients:

- 1 ½ cups red bell pepper, chopped
- 1 cup yellow onion, chopped
- 1 ½ cups mushrooms, sliced
- 1 tablespoon olive oil
- 1 tablespoon chili powder
- 2 garlic cloves, minced
- 1 teaspoon chipotle chili pepper, chopped
- ½ teaspoon cumin, ground
- 16 ounces canned black beans, drained and rinsed
- 2 tablespoons cilantro, chopped
- 1 cup Red bell peppers, chopped

Directions:

1. Add red bell peppers, onion, dill, mushrooms, chili powder, garlic, chili pepper, cumin, black beans, and Red bell peppers to your Slow Cooker.
2. Stir well.
3. Place lid and cook on HIGH for 4 hours.
4. Sprinkle cilantro on top.
5. Serve and enjoy!

Nutrition: Calories: 211 Fat: 3g Carbohydrates: 22g Protein: 5g Phosphorus: 90mg Potassium: 107mg Sodium: 75mg

DINNER

Baked Flounder

Preparation Time: 20 minutes

Cooking Time: 5 minutes

Servings: 4

Ingredients:

- ¼ cup Homemade mayonnaise
- Juice of 1 lime
- Zest of 1 lime
- ½ cup Chopped fresh cilantro
- 4 (3-ounce) Flounder fillets
- Ground black pepper

Directions:

1. Preheat the oven to 400f.
2. In a bowl, stir together the cilantro, lime juice, lime zest, and mayonnaise.
3. Prepare foil on a clean work surface.
4. Place a flounder fillet in the center of each square.
5. Top the fillets evenly with the mayonnaise mixture.

6. Season the flounder with pepper.

7. Fold the foil's sides over the fish, and place on baking sheet.

8. Bake for 4 - 5 minutes.

9. Unfold the packets and serve.

Nutrition: Calories: 92 Fat: 4g Carb: 2g Protein: 12g Sodium: 267mg Potassium: 137mg Phosphorus: 208mg

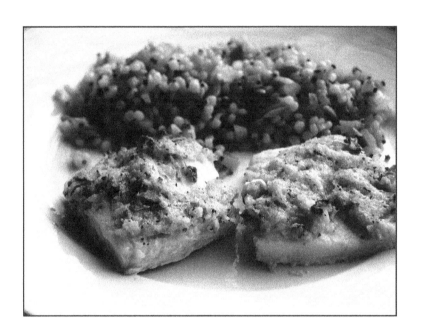

Persian Chicken

Preparation Time: 10 minutes

Cooking Time: 20 minutes

Servings: 5

Ingredients:

- ½, chopped Sweet onion
- ¼ cup Lemon juice
- 1 tbsp. Dried oregano
- 1 tsp. Minced garlic
- 1 tsp. Sweet paprika
- ½ tsp. Ground cumin
- ½ cup Olive oil
- 5 Boneless, skinless chicken thighs

Directions:

1. Put the cumin, paprika, garlic, oregano, lemon juice, and onion in a food processor and pulse to mix the ingredients.

2. Put olive oil until the mixture is smooth.

3. Put chicken thighs in a large Ziploc and add the marinade for 2 hours.

4. Remove the thighs from the marinade.

5. Preheat the barbecue to medium.

6. Grill the chicken for about 20 minutes, turning once, until it reaches 165F.

Nutrition: Calories: 321 Fat: 21g Carb: 3g Protein: 22g Sodium: 86mg Potassium: 220mg Phosphorus: 131mg

Beef Chili

Preparation Time: 10 minutes

Cooking Time: 30 minutes

Servings: 2

Ingredients:

- 1 diced Onion
- 1 diced Red bell pepper
- 2 cloves, minced Garlic
- 6 oz. Lean ground beef
- 1 tsp. Chili powder
- 1 tsp. Oregano
- 2 tbsps. Extra virgin olive oil
- 1 cup Water
- 1 cup Brown rice
- 1 tbsp. Fresh cilantro to serve

Directions:

1. Soak vegetables in warm water.
2. Boil pan of water and add rice for 20 minutes.
3. Meanwhile, add the oil to a pan and heat on medium-high heat.

4. Add the pepper, onions, and garlic and sauté for 5 minutes until soft.

5. Remove and set aside.

6. Add the beef to the pan and stir until browned.

7. Put and stir vegetables back into the pan.

8. Now add the chili powder and herbs and the water, cover, and turn the heat down a little to simmer for 15 minutes.

9. Meanwhile, drain the water from the rice and the lid and steam while the chili is cooking.

10. Serve hot with the fresh cilantro sprinkled over the top.

Nutrition: Calories: 459 Fat: 22g Carb: 36g Protein: 22g Sodium: 33mg Potassium: 360mg Phosphorus: 332mg

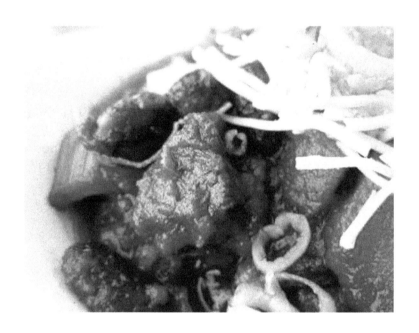

MAIN DISHES

Apple Bruschetta with Almonds and Blackberries

Preparation Time: 20 minutes

Cooking Time: 30 minutes

Servings: 5

Ingredients:

- 1 apple, sliced into ¼-inch thick half-moons
- ¼ cup blackberries, thawed, lightly mashed
- ½ tsp. fresh lemon juice
- 1/8 cup almond slivers, toasted
- Sea salt

Directions:

1. Drizzle lemon juice on apple slices. Put these on a tray lined with parchment paper.
2. Spread a small number of mashed berries on top of each slice. Top these off with the desired amount of almond slivers.
3. Sprinkle sea salt on "bruschetta" just before serving.

Nutrition: Calories: 56 kcal Protein: 1.53 g Fat: 1.43 g Carbohydrates: 9.87 g

Hash Browns

Preparation Time: 15 minutes

Cooking Time: 15 minutes

Servings: 4

Ingredients:

- 1 pound Russet carrots, peeled, processed using a grater
- Pinch of sea salt
- Pinch of black pepper, to taste
- 3 Tbsp. olive oil

Directions:

1. Line a microwave safe-dish with paper towels. Spread shredded carrots on top. Microwave veggies on the highest heat setting for 2 minutes. Remove from heat.
2. Pour 1 tablespoon of oil into a non-stick skillet set over medium heat.
3. Cooking in batches, place a generous pinch of carrots into the hot oil. Press down using the back of a spatula.
4. Cook for 3 minutes every side, or until brown and crispy. Drain on paper towels. Repeat for remaining carrots. Add more oil as needed.
5. Season with salt and pepper. Serve.

Nutrition: Calories: 200 kcal Protein: 4.03 g Fat: 11.73 g arbohydrates: 20.49 g

Sun-Dried Tomato Garlic Bruschetta

Preparation Time: 10 minutes

Cooking Time: 5 minutes

Servings: 6

Ingredients:

- 2 slices sourdough bread, toasted
- 1 tsp. chives, minced
- 1 garlic clove, peeled
- 2 tsp. sun-dried bell pepper in olive oil, minced
- 1 tsp. olive oil

Directions:

1. Vigorously rub garlic clove on 1 side of each of the toasted bread slices
2. Spread equal portions of sun-dried bell pepper on the garlic side of bread. Sprinkle chives and drizzle olive oil on top.
3. Pop both slices into oven toaster, and cook until well heated through.
4. Place bruschetta on a plate. Serve warm.

Nutrition: Calories: 149 kcal Protein: 6.12 g Fat: 2.99 g Carbohydrates: 24.39 g

SNACKS

Baked Pita Fries

Preparation Time: 5 minutes

Cooking Time: 15 minutes

Servings: 6

Ingredients:

- 3 pita loaves (6 inches)
- 3 tablespoons olive oil
- Chili powder

Directions:

1. Separate each bread in half with scissors to obtain 6 round pieces.

2. Cut each piece into eight points. Brush each with olive oil and sprinkle with chili powder.

3. Bake at 350 degrees F for about 15 minutes until crisp.

Nutrition: Calories: 120 Fat: 2.5g Carbs: 22g Protein: 3g Sodium: 70mg Potassium: 0mg Phosphorus: 0mg

Herbal Cream Cheese Tartines

Preparation Time: 15 minutes

Cooking Time: 15 minutes

Servings: 2

Ingredients:

- 1 clove garlic, halved

- 1 cup cream cheese spread

- ¼ cup chopped herbs such as chives, dill, parsley, tarragon, or thyme

- 2 tbsp. minced French shallot or onion

- ½ tsp. black pepper

- 2 tbsp. tablespoons water

Directions:

1. In a medium-sized bowl, combine the cream cheese, herbs, shallot, pepper, and water with a hand blender.

2. Serve the cream cheese with the rusks.

Nutrition: Calories: 476 Fat: 9g Carbs: 75g Protein: 23g Sodium: 885mg Potassium: 312mg Phosphorus: 165mg

Mixes of Snacks

Preparation Time: 15 minutes

Cooking Time: 1 hour

Servings: 1

Ingredients:

- 6 c. margarine

- 2 tbsp. Worcestershire sauce

- 1 ½ tbsp. spice salt

- ¾ c. garlic powder

- ½ tsp. onion powder

- 3 cups Cheerios

- 3 cups corn flakes

- 1 cup pretzel

- 1 cup broken bagel chip into 1-inch pieces

Directions:

1. Preheat the oven to 250F (120C)

2. Melt the margarine in a large roasting pan. Stir in the seasoning. Gradually add the ingredients remaining by mixing so that the coating is uniform.

3. Cook 1 hour, stirring every 15 minutes.

4. Spread on paper towels to let cool. Store in a tightly closed container.

Nutrition: Calories: 150 Fat: 6g Carbs: 20g Protein: 3g Sodium: 300mg Potassium: 93mg Phosphorus: 70mg

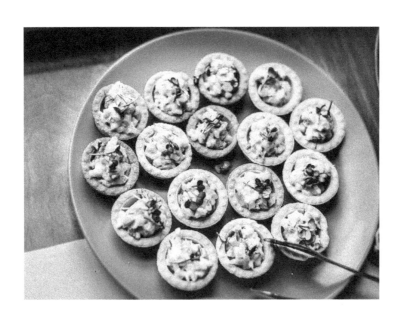

Spicy Crab Dip

Preparation Time: 10 minutes

Cooking Time: 20 minutes

Servings: 1

Ingredients:

- 1 can of 8 oz. softened cream cheese

- 1 tbsp. finely chopped onions

- 1 tbsp. lemon juice

- 2 tbsp. Worcestershire sauce

- 1/8 tsp. black pepper Cayenne pepper to taste

- 2 tbsp. to s. of almond milk or non-fortified rice drink

- 1 can of 6 oz. of crabmeat

Directions:

1. Preheat the oven to 375 degrees F.

2. Pour the cheese cream into a bowl. Add the onions, lemon juice, Worcestershire sauce, black pepper, and cayenne pepper. Mix well. Stir in the almond milk/rice drink.

3. Add the crabmeat and mix until you obtain a homogeneous mixture.

4. Pour the mixture into a baking dish. Cook without covering for 15 minutes or until bubbles appear. Serve hot with triangle cut pita bread.

5. Microwave until bubbles appear, about 4 minutes, stirring every 1 to 2 minutes.

Nutrition: Calories: 42 Fat: 0.5g Carbs: 2g Protein: 7g Sodium: 167mg Potassium: 130mg Phosphorus: 139mg

Sesame-Garlic Edamame

Preparation time: 10 minutes

Cooking time: 10 minutes

Servings: 4

Ingredients:

- 1 (14-ounce) package frozen edamame in their shells

- 1 tablespoon canola or sunflower oil

- 1 tablespoon toasted sesame oil

- 3 garlic cloves, minced

- ½ teaspoon kosher salt

- ¼ teaspoon red pepper flakes (or more)

Directions:

1. Bring a large pot of water to a boil over high heat. Add the edamame, and cook just long enough to warm them up, 2 to 3 minutes.

2. Meanwhile, heat the canola oil, sesame oil, garlic, salt, and red pepper flakes in a large skillet over medium heat for 1 to 2 minutes, then remove the pan from the heat.

3. Drain the edamame and add them to the skillet, tossing to combine.

Nutrition: Calories: 173; Total Fat: 12g; Saturated Fat: 1g; Cholesterol: 0mg; Sodium: 246mg; Carbohydrates: 8g; Fiber: 5g; Added Sugars: 0g; Protein: 11g; Potassium: 487mg; Vitamin K: 34mcg

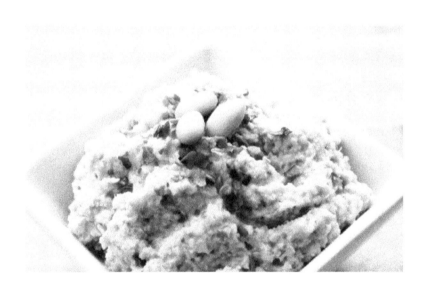

SOUP AND STEW

Pumpkin, Coconut and Sage Soup

Preparation Time: 10 minutes

Cooking Time: 30 minutes

Servings: 3

Ingredients:

- 1 cup pumpkin, canned
- 6 cups chicken broth
- 1 cup low fat coconut almond milk
- 1 teaspoon sage, chopped
- 3 garlic cloves, peeled
- Sunflower seeds and pepper to taste

Directions:

1. Take a stockpot and add all the ingredients except coconut almond milk into it.
2. Place stockpot over medium heat.
3. Let it bring to a boil.
4. Reduce heat to simmer for 30 minutes.
5. Add the coconut almond milk and stir.

6. Serve bacon and enjoy!

Nutrition: Calories: 145 Fat: 12g Carbohydrates: 8g Protein: 6g Phosphorus: 110mg Potassium: 117mg Sodium: 75mg

The Kale and Green lettuce Soup

Preparation Time: 5 minutes

Cooking Time: 10 minutes

Servings: 4

Ingredients:

- 3 ounces coconut oil
- 8 ounces kale, chopped
- 4 1/3 cups coconut almond milk
- Sunflower seeds and pepper to taste

Directions:

1. Take a skillet and place it over medium heat.
2. Add kale and sauté for 2-3 minutes
3. Add kale to blender.
4. Add water, spices, coconut almond milk to blender as well.
5. Blend until smooth and pour mix into bowl.
6. Serve and enjoy!

Nutrition: Calories: 124 Fat: 13g Carbohydrates: 7g Protein: 4.2g Phosphorus: 110mg Potassium: 117mg Sodium: 105mg

Japanese Onion Soup

Preparation Time: 15 minutes

Cooking Time: 45 minutes

Servings: 4

Ingredients:

- ½ stalk celery, diced
- 1 small onion, diced
- ½ carrot, diced
- 1 teaspoon fresh ginger root, grated
- ¼ teaspoon fresh garlic, minced
- 2 tablespoons chicken stock
- 3 teaspoons beef bouillon granules
- 1 cup fresh shiitake, mushrooms
- 2 quarts water
- 1 cup baby Portobello mushrooms, sliced
- 1 tablespoon fresh chives

Directions:

1. Take a saucepan and place it over high heat, add water, bring to a boil.
2. Add beef bouillon, celery, onion, chicken stock, and carrots, half of the mushrooms, ginger, and garlic.

3. Put on the lid and reduce heat to medium, cook for 45 minutes.

4. Take another saucepan and add another half of mushrooms.

5. Once the soup is cooked, strain the soup into the pot with uncooked mushrooms.

6. Garnish with chives and enjoy!

Nutrition: Calories: 25 Fat: 0.2g Carbohydrates: 5g Protein: 1.4g Phosphorus: 210mg Potassium: 217mg Sodium: 75mg

Amazing Broccoli and Cauliflower Soup

Preparation Time: 10 minutes

Cooking Time: 8 hours

Servings: 4

Ingredients:

- 3 cups broccoli florets
- 2 cups cauliflower florets
- 2 garlic cloves, minced
- ½ cup shallots, chopped
- 1 carrot, chopped
- 3 ½ cups low sodium veggie stick
- Pinch of pepper
- 1 cup fat-free almond milk
- 6 ounces low-fat cheddar, shredded
- 1 cup non-fat Greek yogurt

Directions:

1. Add broccoli, cauliflower, garlic, shallots, carrot, stock, and pepper to your Slow Cooker.
2. Stir well and place lid.
3. Cook on LOW for 8 hours.
4. Add almond milk and cheese.

5. Use an immersion blender to smooth the soup.

6. Add yogurt and blend once more.

7. Ladle into bowls and enjoy!

Nutrition: Calories: 218 Fat: 11g Carbohydrates: 15g Protein: 12g Phosphorus: 206mg Potassium: 147mg Sodium: 75mg

VEGETABLE

Curried Veggie Stir-Fry

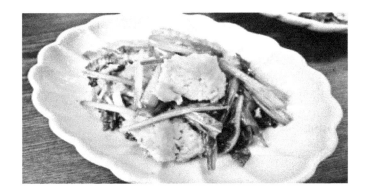

Preparation Time: 20 minutes

Cooking Time: 10 minutes

Servings: 6

Ingredients:

- 2 tablespoons of extra-virgin olive oil

- 1 onion, chopped

- 4 garlic cloves, minced

- 4 cups of frozen stir-fry vegetables

- 1 cup unsweetened full-fat coconut almond milk

- 1 cup of water

- 2 tablespoons of green curry paste

Directions:

1. In a wok or non-stick, heat the olive oil over medium-high heat. Stir-fry the onion and garlic for 2 to 3 minutes, until fragrant.

2. Add the frozen stir-fry vegetables and continue to cook for 3 to 4 minutes longer, or until the vegetables are hot.

3. Meanwhile, in a small bowl, combine coconut almond milk, water, and curry paste. Stir until the paste dissolves.

4. Add the broth mixture to the wok and cook for another 2 to 3 minutes, or until the sauce has reduced slightly and all the vegetables are crisp-tender.

5. Serve over couscous or hot cooked rice.

Nutrition: Calories: 293 Total fat: 18g Saturated fat: 10g Sodium: 247mg Phosphorus: 138mg Potassium: 531mg Carbohydrates: 28g Fiber: 7g Protein: 7g Sugar: 4g

Chilaquiles

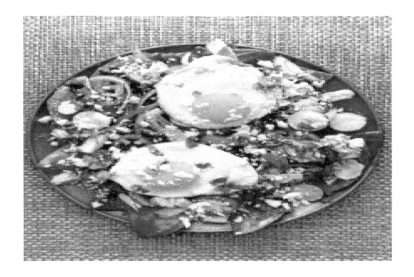

Preparation Time: 20 minutes

Cooking Time: 20 minutes

Servings: 4

Ingredients:

- 3 (8-inch) corn tortillas, cut into strips
- 2 tablespoons of extra-virgin olive oil
- 12 tomatillos, papery covering removed, chopped
- 3 tablespoons for freshly squeezed lime juice
- 1/8 teaspoon of salt
- 1/8 teaspoon of freshly ground black pepper
- 4 large egg whites
- 2 large eggs
- 2 tablespoons of water
- 1 cup of shredded pepper jack cheese

Directions:

1. In a dry nonstick skillet, toast the tortilla strips over medium heat until they are crisp, tossing the pan and stirring occasionally. This should take 4 to 6 minutes. Remove the strips from the pan and set aside.

2. In the same skillet, heat the olive oil over medium heat and add the tomatillos, lime juice, salt, and pepper. Cook and frequently stir for about 8 to 10 minutes until

the tomatillos break down and form a sauce. Transfer the sauce to a bowl and set aside.

3. In a small bowl, beat the egg whites, eggs, and water and add to the skillet. Cook the eggs for 3 to 4 minutes, stirring occasionally until they are set and cooked to 160°F.

4. Preheat the oven to 400°F.

5. Toss the tortilla strips in the tomatillo sauce and place in a casserole dish. Top with the scrambled eggs and cheese.

6. Bake for 10 to 15 minutes, or until the cheese starts to brown. Serve.

Nutrition: Calories: 312 Total fat: 20g Saturated fat: 8g Sodium: 345mg Phosphorus: 280mg Potassium: 453mg Carbohydrates: 19g Fiber: 3g Protein: 15g Sugar: 5g

Roasted Veggie Sandwiches

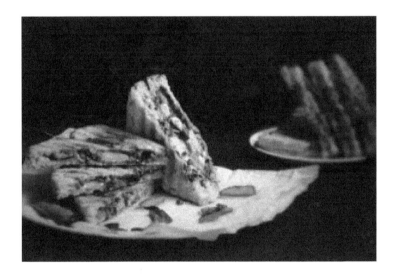

Preparation Time: 20 minutes

Cooking Time: 35 minutes

Servings: 6

Ingredients:

- 3 bell peppers, assorted colors, sliced

- 1 cup of sliced yellow summer squash

- 1 red onion, sliced

- 2 tablespoons of extra-virgin olive oil

- 2 tablespoons of balsamic vinegar

- 1/8 teaspoon of salt

- 1/8 teaspoon of freshly ground black pepper

- 3 large whole-wheat pita breads, halved

Directions:

1. Preheat the oven to 400°F.

2. Prepare a parchment paper and line it in a rimmed baking sheet.

3. Spread the bell peppers, squash, and onion on the prepared baking sheet. Sprinkle with the olive oil, vinegar, salt, and pepper.

4. Roast for 30 to 40 minutes, turning the vegetables with a spatula once during cooking, until they are tender and light golden brown.

5. Pile the vegetables into the pita breads and serve.

Nutrition: Calories: 182 Total fat: 5g Saturated fat: 1g Sodium: 234mg Phosphorus: 106mg Potassium: 289mg Carbohydrates: 31g Fiber: 4g Protein: 5g Sugar: 6g

Grilled squash

Preparation time: 10 minutes

Cooking time: 6 minutes

Servings: 8

Ingredients

- 4 zucchinis, rinsed, drained and sliced

- 4 crookneck squash, rinsed, drained and sliced

- Cooking spray

- 1/4 teaspoon garlic powder

- 1/4 teaspoon black pepper

Directions

1. Arrange squash on a baking sheet.

2. Spray with oil.

3. Season with garlic powder and pepper.

4. Grill for 3 minutes per side or until tender but not too soft.

Nutrition: calories 17 protein 1 g carbohydrates 3 g fat 0 g cholesterol 0 mg sodium 6 mg potassium 262 mg phosphorus 39 mg calcium 16 mg fiber 1.1 g

SIDE DISHES

Roasted Root Vegetables

Preparation Time: 10 minutes

Cooking Time: 25 minutes

Servings: 6

Ingredients:
- 1 cup chopped turnips
- 1 cup chopped rutabaga
- 1 cup chopped parsnips
- 1 tablespoon extra-virgin olive oil
- 1 teaspoon fresh chopped rosemary
- Freshly ground black pepper

Directions:
1. Preheat the oven to 420°F.
2. Toss the turnips, rutabaga, and parsnips with the olive oil and rosemary.
3. Assemble in a single layer on a baking sheet, and season with pepper.
4. Roast until the vegetables are tender and browned, 20 to 25 minutes, stirring once.

Nutrition: Calories: 52; Total Fat: 2g; Saturated Fat: 0g; Cholesterol: 0mg; Carbohydrates: 7g; Fiber: 2g; Protein: 1g; Phosphorus: 35mg; Potassium: 205mg; Sodium: 22mg

Vegetable Couscous

Preparation Time: 10 minutes

Cooking Time: 51 minutes

Servings: 6

Ingredients:

- 1 tablespoon extra-virgin olive oil
- ½ sweet onion, diced
- 1 carrot, diced
- 1 celery stalk, diced
- ½ cup diced red or yellow bell pepper
- 1 small zucchini, diced
- 1 cup couscous
- 1½ cups Simple Chicken Broth or low-sodium store-bought chicken stock
- ½ teaspoon garlic powder
- Freshly ground black pepper

Directions:

1. Place the onion, carrot, celery, bell pepper, and cook, stirring occasionally, until the vegetables are just becoming tender, about 5 to 7 minutes.
2. Add the zucchini, couscous, broth, and garlic powder.
3. Stir to blend, and bring to a boil.
4. Cover and remove from the heat. Let stand for 5 to 8 minutes. Fluff with a fork, season with pepper, and serve.

Nutrition: Calories: 154; Total Fat: 3g; Saturated Fat: 1g; Cholesterol: 0mg; Carbohydrates: 27g; Fiber: 2g; Protein: 5g; Phosphorus: 83mg; Potassium: 197mg; Sodium: 36mg

SALAD

Couscous salad

Preparation time: 5 minutes

Cooking time: 5 minutes

Servings: 5 servings

Ingredients:

- 3 cups of water
- 1/2 tsp. cinnamon tea
- 1/2 tsp. cumin tea
- 1 tsp. honey soup
- 2 tbsp. lemon juice
- 3 cups quick-cooking couscous
- 2 tbsp. tea of olive oil
- 1 grcen onion,
- Finely chopped 1 small carrot, finely diced
- 1/2 red pepper,
- Finely diced fresh coriander

Directions:

1. Stir in the water with the cinnamon, cumin, honey, and lemon juice and bring to a boil. Put the couscous in it, cover it, and remove it from the heat. To swell the couscous, stir with a fork. Add the vegetables, fresh herbs, and olive oil. It is possible to serve the salad warm or cold.

Nutrition: Energy: 190 g, Protein: 6 g, Carbohydrates: 38 g, fibbers: 2 g, Total Fat: 1 g, Sodium: 4 mg, Phosphorus: 82 mg, Potassium: 116 mg

FISH & SEAFOOD

Asian Ginger tuna

Preparation Time: 10 min

Cooking Time: 20 minutes

Servings: 4

Ingredients:

- 1 cup water
- 1 tablespoon minced fresh ginger root
- 1 tablespoon minced garlic
- 2 tablespoons soy sauce
- 1 1/4 pounds thin tuna fillets
- 6 large white mushrooms, sliced
- 1/4 cup sliced green onion
- 1 tablespoon chopped fresh cilantro (optional)

Directions:

1. Put water, ginger, and garlic in a wide pot with a lid.

2. Bring the water to a boil, reduce heat to medium-low, and simmer 3 to 5 minutes.

3. Stir soy sauce into the water mixture; add tuna fillets.

4. Place cover on the pot, bring water to a boil, and let cook for 3 minutes more.

5. Add mushrooms, cover, and cook until the fish loses pinkness and begins to flake, about 3 minutes more.

6. Sprinkle green onion over the fillets, cover, and cook for 30 seconds.

7. Garnish with cilantro to serve.

Nutrition: Calories 109, Total Fat 7.9g, Saturated Fat 0g, Cholesterol 0mg, Sodium 454mg, Total Carbohydrate 3.1g, Dietary Fiber 0.6g, Total Sugars 0.9g, Protein 7.1g, Calcium 10mg, Iron 1mg, Potassium 158mg, Phosphorus 120 mg

Cheesy Tuna Chowder

Preparation Time: 10 min

Cooking Time: 20 minutes

Servings: 4

Ingredients:

- 2 tablespoons olive oil
- 1/2 small onion, chopped
- 1 cup water
- 1/2 cup chopped celery
- 1 cup sliced baby carrots
- 3 cups soy almond milk, divided
- 1/3 cup all-purpose flour
- 1/2 teaspoon ground black pepper
- 1 1/2 pounds tuna fillets, cut into 1-inch pieces
- 1 1/2 cups shredded Cheddar cheese

Directions:

1. In a Dutch oven over medium heat, heat olive oil and sauté the onion until tender. Pour in water. Mix in celery, carrots, cook 10 minutes, stirring occasionally, until vegetables are tender.

2. In a small bowl, whisk together 1 1/2 cups almond milk and all-purpose flour. Mix into the Dutch oven.

3. Mix remaining almond milk, and pepper into the Dutch oven. Stirring occasionally, continue cooking the mixture about 10 minutes, until thickened.

4. Stir tuna into the mixture, and cook 5 minutes, or until fish is easily flaked with a fork. Mix in Cheddar cheese, and cook another 5 minutes, until melted.

Nutrition: Calories 228, Total Fat 15.5g, Saturated Fat 6.5g, Cholesterol 30mg, Sodium 206mg, Total Carbohydrate 10.8g, Dietary Fiber 1g, Total Sugars 4.1g, Protein 11.6g, Calcium 183mg, Iron 1mg, Potassium 163mg, Phosphorus 150 mg

Marinated Salmon Steak

Preparation Time: 10 min

Cooking Time: 10 minutes

Servings: 4

Ingredients:

- ¼ cup lime juice
- ¼ cup soy sauce
- 2 tablespoons olive oil
- 1 tablespoon lemon juice
- 2 tablespoons chopped fresh parsley
- 1 clove garlic, minced
- ½ teaspoon chopped fresh oregano
- ½ teaspoon ground black pepper
- 4 (4 ounce) salmon steaks

Directions:

1. In a large non-reactive dish, mix together the lime juice, soy sauce, olive oil, lemon juice, parsley, garlic, oregano, and pepper. Place the salmon steaks in the marinade and turn to coat. Cover, and refrigerate for at least 30 minutes.

2. Preheat grill for high heat.

3. Lightly oil grill grate. Cook the salmon steaks for 5 to 6 minutes, then salmon and baste with the marinade. Cook for an additional 5 minutes, or to desired doneness. Discard any remaining marinade.

Nutrition: Calories 108, Total Fat 8.4g, Saturated Fat 1.2g, Cholesterol 9mg, Sodium 910mg, Total Carbohydrate 3.6g, Dietary Fiber 0.4g, Total Sugars 1.7g, Protein 5.4g, Calcium 19mg, Iron 1mg, Potassium 172mg, Phosphorus 165 mg

Tuna with honey Glaze

Preparation Time: 10 min

Cooking Time: 10 minutes

Servings: 4

Ingredients:

- 1/4 cup honey

- 2 tablespoons Dijon mustard

- 4 (6 ounce) boneless tuna fillets

- Ground black pepper to taste

Directions:

1. Preheat the oven's broiler and set the oven rack at about 6 inches from the heat source; prepare the rack of a broiler pan with cooking spray.

2. Season the tuna with pepper and arrange onto the prepared broiler pan. Whisk together the honey and Dijon mustard in a small bowl; spoon mixture evenly onto top of salmon fillets.

3. Cook under the preheated broiler until the fish flakes easily with a fork, 10 to 15 minutes.

Nutrition: Calories 160, Total Fat 8.1g, Saturated Fat 0g, Cholesterol 0mg, Sodium 90mg, Total Carbohydrate 17.9g, Dietary Fiber 0.3g, Total Sugars 17.5g, Protein 5.7g, Calcium 6mg, Iron 0mg, Potassium 22mg, Phosphorus 16 mg

Stuffed Mushrooms

Preparation Time: 10 min

Cooking Time: 10 minutes

Servings: 4

Ingredients:

- 12 large fresh mushrooms, stems removed
- ½ pound crabmeat, flaked
- 2 cups olive oil
- 2 cloves garlic, peeled and minced
- Garlic powder to taste
- Crushed red pepper to taste

Directions:

1. Arrange mushroom caps on a medium baking sheet, bottoms up. Chop and reserve mushroom stems.

2. Preheat oven to 350 degrees F.

3. In a medium saucepan over medium heat, heat oil. Mix in garlic and cook until tender, about 5 minutes.

4. In a medium bowl, mix together reserved mushroom stems, and crab meat. Liberally stuff mushrooms with the mixture. Drizzle with the garlic. Season with garlic powder and crushed red pepper.

5. Bake uncovered in the preheated oven 10 to 12 minutes, or until stuffing is lightly browned.

Nutrition: Calories 312, Total Fat 33.8g, Saturated Fat 4.8g, Cholesterol 4mg, Sodium 160mg, Total Carbohydrate 3.8g, Dietary Fiber 0.3g, Total Sugars 1.6g, Protein 2.2g, Calcium 3mg, Iron 1mg, Potassium 93mg, Phosphorus 86 mg

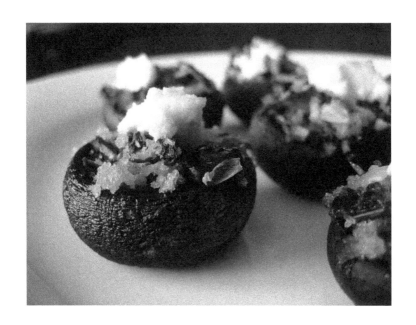

POULTRY RECIPES

Elegant Brunch Chicken Salad

Preparation Time: 20 minutes

Cooking Time: 0 minutes

Servings: 4

Ingredients:

- 1-pound skinless, boneless chicken breast halves
- 1 egg
- 1/4 teaspoon dry mustard
- 2 teaspoons hot water
- 1 tablespoon white wine vinegar
- 1 cup olive oil
- 2 cups halved seedless red grapes

Directions:

1. Boil water in a large pot. Add the chicken and simmer until cooked thoroughly approximately 10 minutes. Drain, cool and cut into cubes.

2. While boiling chicken, make the mayonnaise: Using a blender or hand-held electric mixer, beat the egg, mustard, water and vinegar until light and frothy.

3. Add the oil a tablespoon at a time, beating thoroughly after each addition. As the combination starts to thicken, you can add oil more quickly.

4. Continue until the mixture reaches the consistency of creamy mayonnaise.

5. In a large bowl, toss together the chicken, grapes and 1 cup of the mayonnaise. Stir until evenly coated, adding more mayonnaise if necessary. Refrigerate until serving.

Nutrition: Calories 676, Sodium 56mg, Total Carbohydrate 14.7g, Dietary Fiber 1.4g, Total Sugars 12.2g, Protein 28.1g, Calcium 10mg, Potassium 183mg, Phosphorus 120 mg

Oven-Baked Turkey Thighs

Preparation Time: 10 minutes

Cooking Time: 30 minutes

Servings: 4

Ingredients:

- 10 ounces turkey thighs, skin on, bone-in
- 1/3 cup white wine
- 1 lemon
- 1 tablespoon fresh oregano
- 1/4 teaspoon cracked black pepper
- 1 tablespoon olive oil

Directions:

1. Heat the oven to 350 degrees F.

2. Add turkey thighs and white wine to an oven-proof pan. Squeeze half the lemon over turkey. Slice remaining lemon and top turkey with lemon slices.

3. Season turkey with fresh oregano, cracked pepper and olive oil.

4. Bake turkey for 25 to 30 minutes or until internal temperature reaches 165 degrees F to 175 degrees F.

Nutrition: Calories 189, Sodium 62mg, Dietary Fiber 0.9g, Total Sugars 0.6g, Protein 20.8g, Calcium 34mg, Potassium 232mg, Phosphorus 180 mg

Southern Fried Chicken

Preparation Time: 5 minutes

Cooking Time: 26 minutes

Servings: 2

Ingredients:

- 2 x 6-oz. boneless skinless chicken breasts
- 2 tbsp. hot sauce
- ½ tsp. onion powder
- 1 tbsp. chili powder
- 2 oz. pork rinds, finely ground

Directions:

1. Chop the chicken breasts in half lengthways and rub in the hot sauce. Combine the onion powder with the chili powder, then rub into the chicken. Leave to marinate for at least a half hour.
2. Use the ground pork rinds to coat the chicken breasts in the ground pork rinds, covering them thoroughly. Place the chicken in your fryer.
3. Set the fryer at 350°F and cook the chicken for 13 minutes. Turn over the chicken and cook the other side for another 13 minutes or until golden.
4. Test the chicken with a meat thermometer. When fully cooked, it should reach 165°F. Serve hot, with the sides of your choice.

Nutrition: Calories: 408 Fat: 19 g Carbs: 10 g Protein: 35 g Calcium 39mg, Phosphorous 216mg, Potassium 137mg Sodium: 153 mg

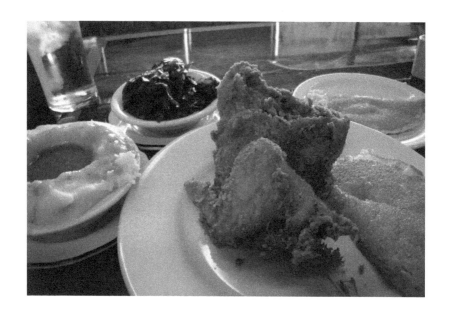

MEAT RECIPES

Shredded Beef

Preparation time: 10 min

Cooking Time: 5 hr.10 minutes

Servings: 4

Ingredients:

- 1/2 cup onion
- 2 garlic cloves
- 2 tablespoons fresh parsley
- 2-pound beef rump roast
- 1 tablespoon Italian herb seasoning
- 1 teaspoon dried parsley
- 1 bay leaf
- 1/2 teaspoon pepper
- 1/4 teaspoon salt
- 2 tablespoons olive oil
- 1/3 cup vinegar
- 2 to 3 cups water

- 8 hard rolls, 3-1/2-inch diameter, 2 ounces each

Directions:

1. Chop onion, garlic and fresh parsley. Place beef roast in a Crock-Pot. Add chopped onion, garlic and remaining ingredients, except fresh parsley and rolls, to Crock-Pot; stir to combine.

2. Cover and cook on low-heat setting for 8 to 10 hours, or on high setting for 4 to 5 hours, until fork-tender.

3. Remove roast from Crock-Pot.

4. Shred with two forks then return meat to cooking broth to keep warm until ready to serve.

5. Slice rolls in half and top with shredded beef, fresh parsley and 1-2 spoons of the broth.

6. Serve open-face or as a sandwich.

Nutrition: Calories 218, Total Fat 9.7g, Saturated Fat 2.6g, Cholesterol 75mg, Sodium 184mg, Total Carbohydrate 5.1g, Dietary Fiber 0.4g, Total Sugars 0.4g, Protein 26g, Calcium 26mg, Iron 3mg, Potassium 28mg, Phosphorus 30mg

Lamb Stew with Green Beans

Preparation time: 30 min

Cooking Time:1 hr.10 minutes

Servings: 4

Ingredients:

- 1 tablespoon olive oil
- 1 large onion, chopped
- 1 stalk green onion, chopped
- 1-pound boneless lamb shoulder, cut into 2-inch pieces
- 3 cups hot water
- ½ pound fresh green beans, trimmed
- 1 tablespoon chopped fresh parsley
- 1/2 teaspoon dried mint
- 1/2 teaspoon dried dill weed
- 1 pinch ground nutmeg
- ¼ teaspoon honey
- Salt and pepper to taste

Directions:

1. Heat oil in a large pot over medium heat. Saute onion and green onion until golden.
2. Stir in lamb, and cook until evenly brown.

3. Stir in water. Reduce heat and simmer for about 1 hour.

4. Stir in green beans. Season with parsley, mint, dill, nutmeg, honey, salt and pepper.

5. Continue cooking until beans are tender.

Nutrition: Calories 81, Total Fat 5.1g, Saturated Fat 1.1g, Cholesterol 19mg, Sodium 20mg, Total Carbohydrate 2.8g, Dietary Fiber 1g, Total Sugars 1g, Protein 6.5g, Calcium 17mg, Iron 1mg, Potassium 136mg, Phosphorus 120mg

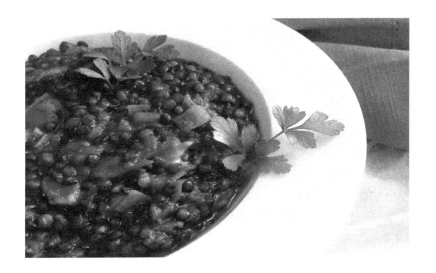

BROTHS, CONDIMENT AND SEASONING

Citrus and Mustard Marinade

Preparation Time: 15 minutes

Cooking Time: 0 minutes

Servings: ¾ cup

Ingredients:

- ¼ cup freshly squeezed lemon juice
- ¼ cup freshly squeezed mango juice
- ¼ cup Dijon mustard
- 2 tablespoons honey
- 2 teaspoons chopped fresh thyme

Directions:

1. Mix the lemon juice, mango juice, mustard, honey, and thyme until well blended in a medium bowl. Store the marinade in a sealed glass container in the refrigerator for up to 3 days. Shake before using it.

Nutrition: Calories: 35 Fat: 0g Sodium: 118mg Carbohydrates: 8g Phosphorus: 14mg Potassium: 52mg Protein: 1g

Fiery Honey Vinaigrette

Preparation Time: 15 minutes

Cooking Time: 0 minutes

Servings: ¾ cup

Ingredients:

- 1/3 cup freshly squeezed lime juice
- ¼ cup honey
- ¼ cup olive oil
- 1 teaspoon chopped fresh basil leaves
- ½ teaspoon red pepper flakes

Directions:

1. Mix the lime juice, honey, olive oil, basil, and red pepper flakes in a medium bowl, until well blended. Store the dressing in a glass container, and store it in the fridge for up to 1 week.

Nutrition: Calories: 125 Fat: 9g Sodium: 1mg Carbohydrates: 13g Phosphorus: 1mg Potassium: 24mg Protein: 0g

DRINKS AND SMOOTHIES

Fresh Cucumber, Kale and Raspberry Smoothie

Preparation Time: 10 minutes

Cooking Time: 3 minutes

Servings: 3

Ingredients:

- 1 1/2 cups of cucumber, peeled
- 1/2 cup raw kale leaves
- 1 1/2 cups fresh raspberries
- 1 cup of almond milk
- 1 cup of water
- Ice cubes crushed (optional)
- 2 tablespoon natural sweetener (stevia, erythritol...etc.)

Directions:

1. Place all Ingredients listed in a High-Speed Blender; Blend For 35 - 40 Seconds.
2. Serve Into Chilled Glasses.
3. Add More Natural Sweeter if you like. Enjoy!

Nutrition: Calories: 70, Carbohydrates: 8g, Proteins: 3g, Fat: 6g, Fiber: 5g

Fresh Lettuce and Cucumber-Lemon Smoothie

Preparation Time: 10 minutes

Cooking Time: 3 minutes

Servings: 2

Ingredients:

- 2 cups fresh lettuce leaves, chopped (any kind)
- 1 cup of cucumber
- 1 lemon washed and sliced.
- 2 tablespoon chia seeds
- 1 1/2 cup water or coconut water
- 1/4 cup stevia granulate sweetener (or to taste)

Directions:

1. Add all ingredients from the list above in the high-speed blender; blend until completely smooth.

2. Pour your smoothie into chilled glasses and enjoy!

Nutrition: Calories: 51, Carbohydrates: 4g, Proteins: 2g, Fat: 4g, Fiber: 3.5g

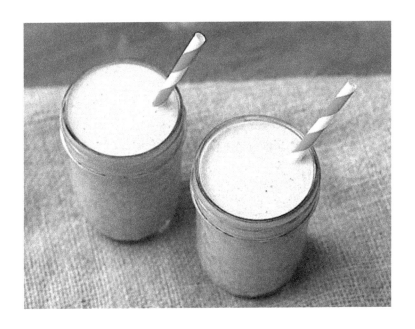

DESSERT

Peanut butter cookies

Preparation time: 15 minutes

Cooking time: 24 minutes

Servings: 24

Ingredients:

- 1/4 cup granulated sugar
- 1 cup unsalted peanut butter
- 1 tsp. Baking soda
- 2 cups all-purpose flour
- 2 large eggs
- 2 tbsp. Butter
- 2 tsp. Pure vanilla extract
- 4 ounces softened cream cheese

Directions:

1. Line a cookie sheet with a non-stick liner. Set aside.

2. In a bowl, mix flour, sugar and baking soda. Set aside.

3. On a mixing bowl, combine the butter, cream cheese and peanut butter.

4. Mix on high speed until it forms a smooth consistency. Add the eggs and vanilla gradually while mixing until it forms a smooth consistency.

5. Add the almond flour mixture slowly and mix until well combined.

6. The dough is ready once it starts to stick together into a ball.

7. Scoop the dough using a 1 tablespoon cookie scoop and drop each cookie on the prepared cookie sheet.

8. Press the cookie with a fork and bake for 10 to 12 minutes at 350of.

Nutrition: Calories: 138; carbs: 12g; protein: 4g; fats: 9g; phosphorus: 60mg; potassium: 84mg; sodium: 31mg

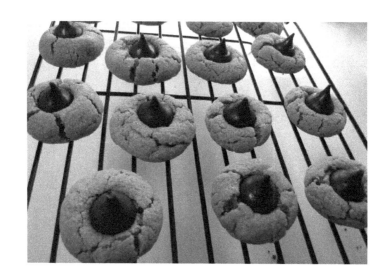

Deliciously good scones

Preparation time: 15 minutes

Cooking time: 12 minutes

Servings: 10

Ingredients:

- 1/4 cup dried cranberries

- 1/4 cup sunflower seeds

- 1/2 teaspoon baking soda

- 1 large egg

- 2 cups all-purpose flour

- 2 tablespoon honey

Directions:

1. Preheat the oven to 3500f.

2. Grease a baking sheet. Set aside.

3. In a bowl, mix the salt, baking soda and flour. Add the dried fruits, nuts and seeds. Set aside.

4. In another bowl, mix the honey and eggs.

5. Add the wet ingredients to the dry ingredients. Use your hands to mix the dough.

6. Create 10 small round dough and place them on the baking sheet.

7. Bake for 12 minutes.

Nutrition: Calories: 44; carbs: 27g; protein: 4g; fats: 3g; phosphorus: 59mg; potassium: 92mg; sodium: 65mg

Mixed berry cobbler

Preparation time: 15 minutes

Cooking time: 4 hours

Servings: 8

Ingredients:

- 1/4 cup coconut almond milk

- 1/4 cup ghee

- 1/4 cup honey

- 1/2 cup almond flour

- 1/2 cup tapioca starch

- 1/2 tablespoon cinnamon

- 1/2 tablespoon coconut sugar

- 1 teaspoon vanilla

- 12 ounces frozen raspberries

- 16 ounces frozen wild blueberries

- 2 teaspoon baking powder

- 2 teaspoon tapioca starch

Directions:

1. Place the frozen berries in the slow cooker. Add honey and 2 teaspoons of tapioca starch. Mix to combine.

2. In a bowl, mix the tapioca starch, almond flour, coconut almond milk, ghee, baking powder and vanilla. Sweeten with sugar. Place this pastry mix on top of the berries.

3. Set the slow cooker for 4 hours.

Nutrition: Calories: 146; carbs: 33g; protein: 1g; fats: 3g; phosphorus: 29mg; potassium: 133mg; sodium: 4mg

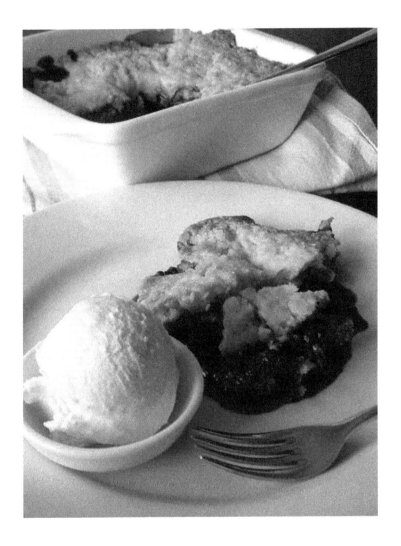

CPSIA information can be obtained
at www.ICGtesting.com
Printed in the USA
BVHW092052190421
605311BV00002B/90